In the Extra Years

poetry by

Roger Sippl

For more information about this title or to order other books
and/or electronic media, contact the publisher:

TwoSistersWriting.com
18530 Mack Avenue, Suite 166
Grosse Pointe Farms, MI 48236

ISBN:
978-1-945875-96-0 (Paperback)
978-1-945875-97-7 (eBook)

Printed in the United States of America

Cover and Interior design: Van-garde Imagery

To our Elizabeth,
my mate for life,
thanks for helping to save me
and for taking care of me.

Contents

Contents

Preface

THIS BOOK IS ABOUT how I spent the rest of my life after I survived, at age 19, Hodgkin's Lymphoma, a type of cancer that, at the time, only gave me a 20 percent chance of living further. This book is poetry. Therefore, it doesn't detail everything I did. Many events in my past just don't make good poetry.

I took three companies public, and while it got me the Golden Hat Trick Award from my underwriter, Cristina Morgan, all that business stuff just isn't very lyrical, although I suppose someday I should try to make it so. But there is a little factoid that does make for a good story, if not a poem. Once, for a week-long party with my friends in the Caribbean, I chartered a cruise ship.

It only had 50 staterooms, so it was a small cruise ship, as cruise ships go. Chartering it was motivated by the desire, when I thought I was dying, to just go to the beach with my friends. When I thought I was going to lose them all, all at once, that was my number one thought. Years after my cancer treatment, I had some success in the software business and I realized I never took that time to hang out with my friends on a sunny day in the sand. After the third IPO, I decided I was probably at the peak of things, so I declared it to be "The Year of Roger" and took my friends on this trip "to the beach" – which became "The Year of Roger Cruise" complete with logowear, fireworks one night, a toga party another, and the inevitable martini-tasting contest with talent show put on completely by my guests.

I did things like that in the extra years. Perhaps all my life I was that way in my mind, but after cancer, I lived it—too confident, impulsive and too willing to forget about the consequences of failure. Cancer made me more sure that nothing good was going to happen for me unless I made it happen, and further, bad things were definitely going to happen, no matter what, so I better enjoy my life right now before it's too late.

Whether you call it a good attitude or a bad attitude, it made for a wonderful life. In my next book, I'll fill in the blanks between the poems with prose, explain what was going on when I wrote each poem, and what I meant to say by writing it, to the extent I know. But for now, I'll leave you with just the poems, and you'll have the luxury of exactly your own interpretation.

Please let me know any thoughts you have on any of the poems, or the whole collection, at roger@sipmac.com.

Thanks for reading.

Roger Sippl
Silicon Valley, California
2021

Having Cancer

The Sweater

The doctors tell me the main tumor
in my chest is the size of a softball.
She uses a double strand of yarn

and thin knitting needles so the arms and walls
to cover my chest and back will be thick.
There are more in my bronchial system,

my neck, below my diaphragm, and maybe
in my spleen. The sweater will warm me
even in the wind. She had to do Catholic

Penance, a mother's labor, she repeats
non-stop clicks with yarn, mostly acrylic,
so it can't be eaten and

will never decay. She says it is her
fault. She should have stopped me from
sneaking onto that stupid golf course at night, swimming

with mosquitoes, diving the black lake for lost balls
through industrial fertilizer and green dyes, as if
she knows what caused my lymph node cancer

when no one else does. She tries to cure me, feels
my forehead, clicks the needles together again
and again until her fingers hurt and wrists ache

and she can hardly stand up from sitting so long.
So I tell her that leaves on trees blow left
then right, some rattle and flip,

some move hardly at all, yet some are first to fall
to the ground. I tell her the sweater
is coming along great as she watches me lose

weight lying in bed. The needles click as she approaches
another threshold of pain
that relieves her.

The Rest of Them

The small animals are only
made of salt crystals rolled
into spheres, imperfect,
blowing from right to left,

north to south, across the freeway
approaching the entrance
to the Dumbarton Bridge
which spans the miles of estuary

of lower San Francisco Bay.
They blow, pause, swirl and re-blow,
dashing across the road terrified
by cars with tires that flatten some of them,
        uncaring.

Truly, only salt and foam blown from the protein
and brackish mix on the surface of the bay—
water blown into ripples, then waves
that the wind pushes to trip over

the shallow mud flat near San Jose,
their tops gusting off
into this tumbling mist that dries instantly
leaving behind, in mid-air, the exoskeletons

of these life forms that have shed
that surface for balling up to eddy then rush
across these streets that separate
salt marsh from open fields.

Some give themselves up —
hope expiring, like me, on my way

Having Cancer

to Stanford University Medical Center
feeling sorry for myself with solid tumors,

not feeling the attempted cure supposedly
underway, doubting it entirely, letting myself cry
while changing to the fast lane to pass my thoughts
as I run over those few that I can, worrying

about the rest of them,
escaping to the other side of the freeway,
floating and flowing through the open fields,
blowing out of sight.

Dear Mr. Harvey

Thank you for your note of three years ago,
and thank you for being my AP English teacher.
I enjoyed the course.
Yes, as a junior at Berkeley
I was diagnosed with cancer. Your offer of help
was much appreciated.

I write to you now because
no matter how your day is going,
no matter what mood you are in
I think everyone needs a good cry
once in a while, and this is that time.

It's not bad news,
it'll be a happy cry.

In those three years I have not relapsed.
I have gone from a twenty percent chance
to an eighty percent chance of survival.
I think I'm going to make it.

I had to stay in school to keep my student health insurance,
because it was the only coverage I had,
but I was able to do that. Although it was torture,
and took five years of college in total,
healthy, then sick, then recovering,
I got my degree, and I now have a job,

and a girlfriend,
and she loves me.

In the Extra Years

I was scheduled to die young
but I didn't, so, in the extra years,
knowing for sure that you never know,
I have needed to live an extra-ordinary life.

In the extra years, each day arrived like a new lover,
exciting to touch, beside me for all the fun,
holding me as it got rough, caressing me
to be my best, for her, for our romance.

I built a house on a cliff, the Pacific on three sides with
midnight storm waves booming white water. A calm rocky
beach at sunrise, where, among the cold kelp, in the extra years,
I dived for abalone to fry in garlic butter, breakfast for my friends.

Leading people, leading leaders,
I earned a way to live a life based on living,
unafraid, hard to bluff, and I surprised
them all by writing poetry – they never knew.

Truly knowing what I truly knew, I could have worn white robes,
walked on hot coals and explained God to everyone
willing to listen. Maybe I did, in my way,
in the extra years, always looking back at that day

the doctor told my 19-year-old self,
"You have Hodgkin's Disease,"
and I asked,
"What is it?"

Just a Test

I'm radioactive now
and emitting positrons,
which are very small but
large enough to make a dot
on a film or sensor somewhere
inside this machine.

It's just a test
to see if my cancer has come back,
or perhaps a new cancer has formed.

The trace of dots
will look like me,
and if none of my lymph nodes
light up from the hot sugar water
now in my blood, homing the nuclear-rigged
glucose to any
over-active cancer nodes,
then I'll be fine.

Bridgehampton

Road-Side Farm Stand

Triple-ripe peaches,
not so ripe as to be mushy,
but even chilled
the firm flesh gushes
the sugar built from recent days
of moist sunshine.

Can we have just this—
take just the goodness,
and ignore the quick-onset arthritis
of a dear friend, or
the just-dead husband of another?

In Bridgehampton can't we just be
on vacation and not be in the real?
Maybe not.

Sweet Corn

Corn is different.
Sweet and white,
so, boil water in a pot at home now
as Mom stops at a field
owned by someone she knows
but doesn't care for,
flashes into the rows,
at least five deep
to get past the cow corn
and right back out
with the good stuff.
It has only one hour
to get into and out of the pot
(more fruit stands
but no time
to stop)
and be eaten with butter, pepper
and salt—

only that sweetness,
short time in the mouth,
so tightly binds our memories
to these last few weeks of summer.

Mecox Beach

Girls at the beach
show off their new tops
ostensibly playing Frisbee
hoping the boys will join.

The boys play baseball
on the radio
hoping the girls
will come over
and pretend to listen
together with them.

Salt Water

Salt water cures everything so
when her husband died suddenly
from that heart attack which
was totally unforeseen she
needed to go into the ocean
and float.

He was funny, fixed her drinks
and lived with her for over thirty years
as her husband and father of her two children.

So the cure is the gulf stream,
swimming in it and now floating,
looking up at the clouds moving
in the late afternoon sky,
such that her head is far enough back
that the rest of her body rises

until she can see her toes sticking up.
Keeping her ears yet in the water
she doesn't have to hear anything
but the sounds of the undersea.

Black

Walking in the black
home from the bar
because the streets are not lit
and the taxis don't run
after midnight.

The Light

When the sun is low,
whether rising or setting,
its light reflects off the dunes
and the grasses growing up through the top of them,
imprinting all that detail into your eyes.

The Geese

The Canadian geese are getting booed
by locals and tourists
from Montauk to Queens
because of the meaning
that flies overhead—
summer is now over.

It's the week when the children's camps
all along the East Coast have come to an end,
but school hasn't started yet,
and so, it's family week,
when anyone with any connection to Long Island is here,
remembering that the huge squawking Canadian Geese
really do fly from Canada to Florida,
right over New York,
definitively marking the end of the season.

The V-shape of the flock
has the children asking,
"Why do they fly that way?" and,
"How do they know?"

You think about explaining that each bird
feels the up-and-down of the sinusoidal vortex
twirling off the outside wingtip of
the bird ahead and to the side
and each bird adjusts its position
in the formation, constantly,
to ride, just a little, on the up-wash
it senses rolling off its flock-mate.

But then you simply answer,
"Because nature loves a graceful ending."

Cuba

Havana Club

When in Havana, you drink Havana Club straight,
sipping, swirling high in the light, tasting the balance
of caramel and oak from twelve years' captive in cask.

The rum master does not apologize for the numbness
on our tongues or for his four-pocket shirt,
but he pulls our attention to the warmth and the long finish.

He explains all rum is a blend.
This distillery, born in the 1800's, is,
"historically, the best blender

of the soil, the sun and the brown sugar of Cuba
together with the jazz drums, salsa dance
and the unabashed friendliness of the Cubans."

We drink our large samples and try, but fail, to blow off the excess alcohol,
and before long our host smiles to tell us
that we have, together, "woken up the Devil."

No Religion

Religious beliefs and practices
were banned by *la revolucion*
as the opium of the people.

So, there is no reason for the horse and buggy, bouncing along
on the farm, no Amish discipline outlawing the truck,
just the onerous two-hundred-and-forty-percent import tax
and the complete lack of personal wealth. Also,
a Sputnik gas station in Camaquey is a rare sighting,
in that town of the pre-soviet sugar barons. Maybe the cane farmers
use horses instead of trucks because horses manufacture themselves,
and need no government import permit.
But no, God did not forbid new trucks or tractors in Cuba.

The Godliness of Fidel and Che, though, is taught in the schools.
Other than those songs and stories of victory and salvation
the people mostly choose no God of their own
because, by law, there is none.

Yet the Pope came to visit
and was allowed in for some reason.
An unknown number of people re-found a Spanish faith,
or, secretly, their Santeria slave voodoo,
which hundreds of years ago was disguised to look like Catholicism,
so it would not be banned, even then. Now
some churches have opened again for business,

allowed perhaps because there is an empty and collapsing church
in every town square, with internal artwork looking for a purpose,
or perhaps because Karl Marx also wrote:

> *Religion is the sigh of the oppressed creature,*
> *the heart of a heartless world,*
> *and the soul of soulless conditions.*

Between the Mangroves

There is often a reef between the clumps of mangroves,
maybe a few acres per island of trees with the roots
that begin latticing before entering the water.

Sometimes the shallow bottom between these patches is sand
with beds of sea grass. Sometimes there is coral.
Without the mangroves, the baby lobsters, goliath groupers,

and the endemic species have no place to grow up
with protection from the bigger reef fish.
The mangroves are the nursery, the only nursery.

The endemic species happen because the island itself
is an ecosystem, and the shallows just around its terrestrial edges
are private. The suction of the island keeps the organisms

mixing their gene pools close to home,
creating the Cuban golden basslet, one-inch long,
yellow with a splash of purple and black,

and keeps the majority of Cubans still hoping that
the Muse of Socialism is beautiful, with the flowing hair
they see in the history books of Greece and Rome,

and she is not the hollow and stern stepmother
living with them.

Mating for Life

Everyday

All through each long day
our nightgowns hug each other
on the bedroom hook.

The Lover's Etiquette

When two lovers have a box
containing two chocolates
of different shapes,
colors, textures or aromas

The Lover's Etiquette states
that each should bite
off half, melt
the hard shell with

the heat of the mouth,
and tongue that together
with the ganache
inside until the raspberry

or coconut or rum
or coffee is confirmed
and then offer
the other half.

Simple Love Formula

Love
is good
and
hate
is bad.

Since we have our love
all we have to do
is simply decide not to hate.

We can date others,
no problem—
this can work,
and we'll prove it.

    Maybe this could have worked,
    I don't know. I haven't the science
    to know the theoretical chance.
    But it clearly
    did not work.

        There is a different way,
        a simple love formula that we did not try.
        Find your love and stay with her.
        Do everything
        to be with her, until
        you die.

Love Locks

Was he locking his bike or locking his love
when he quickly secured the three-foot-long bicycle lock
to the Louvre Bridge, the *Pont des Arts*?

His lock sits among the short locks of those mated for life—
the ones that can take a fat-caliber, high-speed,
metal-jacketed bullet straight through the tumblers—and hold.

Was he pleading for latitude, some leash,
both love and freedom, and did he understand
his request?

The saddest lover sang, "freedom only helps you say goodbye,"
and knowing this, every true lover that was ever on the bridge
believes all the love songs, and they walk across slowly, with no car, no bike,

just their lover,
and they throw the key
as far down river as they can.

My Family

He Likes Primary Colors

He likes primary colors
but he knows when Mommy is dressed up pretty.

He smiles badly for pictures
unless he actually thinks something is funny
or is tickled and he's in the mood for that.

He's tough, and doesn't mind bleeding a little bit
to do something he feels is important,
like practicing with his new skateboard
on the street, which is rougher than the tennis court.

He is four, almost five,
and when he is tired he needs his sleep,
but is sometimes too tired to fall asleep without the help that I give him,
rubbing and rocking, and something soft to hold or stroke,
to relax his mind—put him somewhere else,
outside the womb, but almost as safe, in the real world,
which he is learning about at a desperate rate.

He Takes Chances

In a long slow dance exhausted
shuffling around the room, moving in
a circle, while twisting
with my arms around myself
I hug my baby that is not
there, being watched by the
stuffed animals that waited
for him to be born fourteen and a half years ago.

He is at his six-week-long
"wilderness camp" in our American Siberia
supposedly learning what his life with me
did not transfer to his working brain.

He takes chances.
Good or bad he takes chances.

And he must learn the difference.

He's broken just the things
I cannot fix
and in his subconscious he'll fight
the demons that he built
so that he can defeat them on his own.

He takes chances.
Good or bad he takes chances.

And he must learn the difference.

While on his "survival course"
his younger brother and sister will not understand
why he had to live long enough in the ice

to find himself, and then go away
to a therapeutic boarding school
for an infinite eighteen months.

We will have to get them a kitten.

He takes chances.
Good or bad he takes chances.

And he must learn the difference.

Heavenly Whispers

Heavenly Whispers

The two nurses were leaning over me
as I lay flat in the hospital bed
looking up at them arguing against each other
about which way the two differently-colored wires,
one green and one red,
should be inserted
into the electrical ports on
the small black box with the battery in it.
The wires ran straight to my heart.

(This is done after open-heart surgery—two pacing leads
are left touching your heart and they trace out into the air
so, if your heart stops beating
after closure
this little box with the nine-volt
can be used for the jump start
instead of the big external paddles,
which are crude.)

"The red wire goes into the port on the right side—yes?"

"Yes, but forward? Which way? How do you know?"

I was almost seeing the full colors of the nurses
and the room elements again when I started talking,
"Ladies, let's wait for the doctor now—I'm fine."

They didn't shock me, since I was clearly awake,
but I stopped short of telling them about the white.
Everything had faded to white, as if peroxide had cut loose
and my brain had sponged it all as it completely bleached.

I couldn't hear the alarms at the nurse's station
or in my room when I was out, but I am sure

they were loudly alerting
about the flat line.

I could barely hear
the guy dressed in white holding the white clipboard,
talking too softly, whispering, and
saying, "Walk toward the light" or
did he say, "Walk toward the right"—you don't want to
make a mistake like that at such an important juncture.
The white was welcome at first,
blissful in its simplicity and resolution
but seriously, I had to force myself to think,
to ask the question,

"Do I really want this to be over?"

The Pier

The children who visit enjoy
the Heavenly Whispers Pier.
There isn't anything on it—
it isn't like the Santa Monica Pier
with a merry-go-round and
roller coaster along with
stands for corn dogs and lemonade
or a frozen banana.
It's a small and simple pier.

But piers are special
all by themselves.

They are a way to visit another world.

You are on land
and then with just a little walking
you are suddenly in the aquatic world
and have a masterful point of view.

> From the end of the Heavenly Whispers pier
> I could see my surgery,
> which was no big deal,
> but was needed to fix the valve
> that was damaged by the radiation,
> absorbed more than forty years prior
> to treat Hodgkin's Lymphoma,
> stage IIIB no less—and
> yes, B was worse than A—not
> to mention the emotional scars from
> the chemotherapy, the unfindable,
> untouchable ones.

The children catch tadpoles
using dip nets and put them
into one-time pickle jars
that become the aquariums
of scientific discovery and demonstration.

They explain to their grandparents,
our residents,
how some of the pollywogs
have formed legs,
have shorter tails
and are becoming frogs,
because that is what some older kid
told them.

The children are amazed at the changes.
Our residents are not so amazed,
knowing change as they do, but
they are charmed by the children's
emotion of fascination
and they try to remember when that was last true
in themselves.

The Neighbor Lady

Evelyn has been sick for a while
but fighting a "good fight" and holding up well,
two small houses down

the cul-de-sac from my
one-bedroom free-standing unit here at
Heavenly Whispers.

Yesterday she made it to group lunch.
I told her I would visit this morning
and her always-round eyes

opened a little more than
they usually do.
She stuttered to a smile

and said, "Fine!"
So, this is no time for the usual things to say.
She is leaving soon.

I won't be shy this time.
I won't talk around the edges.
I might not talk at all.

When I arrive I look at her face and see that she is looking at me
knowing why my hand on her cheek is so tender,
and then even in the stupor from her new favorite drug,

the opiate, she sees
that I am selfishly thinking of my own
old cancer, long gone, but with my own death

right behind hers anyway.
She is lying in bed,
under a sheet and a comforter

filled with down feathers,
bagged in a cotton duvet,
her head on big pillows.

She still has a husband
and before he fell and broke his hip,
or vice versa, we played golf.

He's in the Heavenly Whispers
Assisted Living Building after his replacement
surgery, not moving much on his own.

But she and I have always understood each other,
having more common interests, especially musical theater,
dated each other in high school and both being atheists.

So, I take his place right now
in one role that he could never serve
anyway—to help her reflect—

because he's still looking forward
to all kinds of things, his mind foolishly random
and busy, not focused, like mine.

She slides a tube across the night stand toward me
and I squeeze her sweet fruit-punch morphine gel
under my own tongue,

not to join her in her death,
but to take the journey
far enough with her, a companion,

    as back then, with the summer joint and
    small cooler of ice and dark Dos Equis, the corn chips
    and the salty beach in the night time.

The grunion were running, scheduled
to flap their bodies against the wet sand
laying eggs and fertilizing them at midnight.

We walked from the car through the black air
to our secret sand dune, laid out
the army blanket and I opened a beer while she lit up,

expertly, in the welcome orange light
of the match, drawing the smoke in,
sharing and laughing unseen by anyone

and invisible to each other,
settling just in time
to see the fish.

They became land animals temporarily,
as a wave retreated exposing their plan
in the surprise light of a large and quickly-rising moon

that broke the horizon full,
climbing up and to the right,
away from the dunes and away from us. But today

I'm on top of the sheet, on top of the duvet
and its feathers that wrap her, bundling her
in her confidence so she'll be ready for her transition.

She feels like a solid mass
that I can lie next to, again
my head touching hers on the pillow, one arm comfortably

across her chest, my hand cupped on her shoulder.
My mind finally numbs warm
with the forbidden rush of our new drug

starting to circulate through my own body, someone
who is not on the hospice protocol, but rather
part of it.

She whispers, "This is the one real thing you've done.
Perhaps knowing you was worth the aggravation
after all."

Young Love

Young Love

Then my face was close to hers,
my first true date, at the end of the evening.
I was looking straight at her and knew she
was looking at me.

The freckles on her nose and to the sides
now showed, but soft
was all I could think when my cheek
pressed hers and I felt sorry about my new whiskers.

Pulling back four inches her preparations were now clear—
attempted bedroom eyes, thin lines of body art
all of it darker than I saw
just before English class when I asked her out.

Her shoulder-length hair swayed and carried the fragrance
of her teenage shampoo. The clean shine of it across my face,
as she nuzzled me with her neck, made me drunk enough of its common flowers
to transcend being a boy—and never recover as an adult.

Not since babyhood
had I been bound so tightly to the scent
of a woman.
Something was gone, something new.

Her slickered lips on mine,
and then more. It was my first time kissing
on her porch, but not hers, and I had to decide
if I cared.

Kissing on the Cliff

Do you remember the moist air?
In the black night we couldn't see the plants
on the ground, near the edge,
until our eyes adjusted.
Then you would look for the stars and
later I'd point out the white glow from the surf
when a wave broke.

So Many Stars

Henry Mancini opened the show, and played piano
with a full orchestra of Hollywood studio musicians,
some brass, but mostly violins, cellos and bass,
pouring out his movie-sweet love songs,
filling the outdoor Greek Amphitheater with clear simple syrup.

The glycerin of *Moon River's* major chords,
found a spillway down the bluffs to the flat river-delta floor
and fingered up the streets
to cover the point lights, people and cars
of Los Angeles with this studio-commissioned
theme that he played from his author's memory,
convincing me that he wrote it for himself after all.
The ooze deepened, too clear to be seen and so dense
that it slowed down time in the LA basin
and the surrounding hills.

Lani Hall was next, singing with Sergio Mendez
and his jazz band, seductively in her native-looking role,
as if she were eighteen again, unmarried, back in a Brazilian bar
looking and longing for a new lover.
She sang *Mas Que Nada* synchronously alongside a long-legged Latin beauty,
both in the same black, one-shoulder-free, one-strap dresses,
attacking each note together in one doubled voice.

> You sat next to me at that concert
> above the big valley of former farmland,
> southern, warm-night lovely, young in love and locked
> in that moment for sure
> as music was your primary medium.

> You could stretch your own songs from
> high alto to true soprano and I wished to hear

your full, slow and rounded tones with no separate vibrations
revealed by your shy captive voice.

Lani finally sang *So Many Stars*—

Which one to choose,
which way to go, how can I tell how will I know, out of, oh,
so many stars, so many stars?

And so many stars
were, my dear, offering above
all futures, but Lani sang of our just one choice—
so, given the breadth of our future and our velocity going through it

our chances together were humble and slight.

We looked up at our real stars from within her song,
not stoned, too young to drink even,
interlacing fingers, my arm inside of yours,
and you pressed against me like a drug, my drug, and
the mental image of the above shutter-clicked for my lifetime
of not knowing whether to forever choose
or to take the risk, with time slowed down as it was,
to tease the fabric of the black part of the sky into strings,
and use more than one thread
to choose more than one star,
including the one that would come back to you
singing your choices
and chance to find you, after all,

with some version of me.

Laura,

We were in Santa Cruz a year ago,
you told me you met him
I turned on that beach facing you
damn it, Laura, I grabbed your elbows hard.
I turned on you on that beach
damn it, Laura, damn it.

In Santa Cruz, in the evening,
there was an old sailing vessel aground on the beach,
its bow intact but jammed into that high
bank of sand, the stern only touched by
the ends of the waves. Bearded men in rain coats
shoveled sand carefully, bulldozers sent out cables
to the mast, the black ship with white
windows and orange light in the cabins
could not be moved. Several days later
the ship was freed and it sailed well away
from the land where in very cold water
it sank all the way to the ocean's floor
where a large rock formation broke it
in half, the stern slid upright onto the sand,
the bow scraped against the rock and tipped
over as it fell to be broken by the surge
cracking wood against the rocks, until
all of the parts were scattered by the moving water
and one or two washed ashore.

But now in this dark and crowded room with pulsing jazz
I see the cufflink of the man with whom you are drinking.
I stand up and walk to the men's room,
re-comb part of my hair and undo the second button on my shirt.
I walk out into the light of the exit and
as I watch the back of your neck he glances up at me.
I walk home and go to sleep.

To Walk with Laura

Each foot had eight stitches
from the bipedal lymphangiography.
The tumors in my chest
were so large and numerous

they thought there would be more
below my diaphragm,
and there were. A scalpel
cut the tops of my feet.

I lay still on the table—
one-inch incisions allowing sterile
salad oil to percolate
up my lymph vessels

paralleling my leg veins,
from feet into abdomen,
this contrast agent lighting up
the over-sized nodes, now less dense

than everything else on the x-ray.
The stitches made it hard to walk
on the sand, and to walk with Laura
I had to walk on the sand

and I had to walk with Laura. We would
watch the sunsets on the beach together when
we were in love, but we weren't in love
anymore. Maybe Jim?

But she never said anything special
about him, which I didn't want to hear
anyway. Of all the drugs offered
she was my self-medication.

In exchange for quiet shivering
from the pain of clawing the dry sand
I heard about arguments with Jim, how he made
her cry, and how this visit was a complication.

We made it to bed, her cotton nightgown
smooth where I lay my head on
the flannel stretched over her chest—salve
and salvation for my brain

thinking of the radiation still burning
deep into my chest and the seven months
to come, chemotherapy poison dripping
into my veins, needle in the back of my left hand.

I had to find the line, the line
between giving up and giving up entirely.
I did give up on her
as any source of refuge,

and everything else Laura,
but I did not give up on my own slim chance
alone—passing from her, and that night,
into adulthood.

Burning Man

Why Burn the Man?

The seventy-thousand people
that have come to the Burning Man Festival
with me on this alkaline dry lake bed
are creating more than an art party.

We have pre-selected ourselves as those willing
to be the most accepting
souls of other souls and the most
willing to try to evolve.

The brochure says we choose to practice
radical inclusionism,
radical self-reliance
and eight other principles
that make a person the best.
Giving not selling,
respecting not trampling
but we lock our bikes.

Is the temporary utopia
the real gimmick?
Not the thirty-foot high armadillo
art car, hundred-tit march, non-judgmental twister yoga
or the voting booth for God?

They take a census at Town Center
to ask, "Why does this work?"
Why do people camp on this piece of land
that has been shown to be
uninhabitable, coming from San Francisco
but also London, Lisbon and Melbourne?

Feeding the community for free
cannot last long. A quarter-billion dollars

of resources are spent
to try to find the best of man and woman,
sustain the perfectly simple human
for just one week. But we can't
go any longer. We
know that. We have to
burn him down.

The Release

At Burning Man we build things
and then burn them until there is nothing.

The Man, of course, is the center of this,
but the more personal sub-centers are where
we do what we came to do—
get the release.

You write two notes on sheets from a pad
of lineless paper, thumbtack them to
the pine pagoda, say goodbye to Mom,
and let Dad know that you hated him for a reason.

You do this now because you've heard
that the building burns
in hundred-foot flames
tonight.

Cattle

Los Angeles, 1862

With the light of his new oil lamp Governor Stanford
reads the weather report in the Star:
"On Tuesday last the sun made its appearance.
The phenomenon lasted several minutes
and was witnessed by a great number of persons."

It is rumored that the once flourishing settlement
of Anaheim is completely destroyed,
and the few buildings that marked the
collective center for the ranchos of Los Angeles
have been overturned or broken apart.

When the flooding began
the farmers gathered their turkeys into a shelter.
Now the water is very deep and the cattle
are difficult to shelter. When they are located
they are seen panicked to stampede
although their hooves just touch the mud.
They keep trying to run until finally they disappear.

Dana Point, 1835

In the warm morning fog
a New England sailing vessel
carefully ties to short pilings in the cove.
As several men hoist a long boat
they hear the hollering of dying cattle
and the crack of sledge hammers.
Like heavy carpets the wet skins fall from the cliff.
The men are careful not to overload the boat.

Santa Catalina Island, 1864

They hear the random clanging of a small bell,
the Union soldiers row from their cruiser,
they climb the cliff to find the cattle,
the cattle that are thin like goats.

The vegetation of the island is sparse
but wild currants, mashed cactus juices
and occasional sea lions could support a man
or a group of men; only officers leave the ship.

Two uniformed marksmen fall to their right knees
and aim at the cow's forehead. The animal falls
while still chewing something. They tow the cow
to the ship in a boat of its own.

While unloading, the boat capsizes.
The cow sinks into very clear black water.

Losing Dave

Don't Try to Find Me

Dave, it was a good movie.
Your daughter liked it and your wife as well.
They both thought the original
Mary Poppins was the movie of their generation
but this was good.

I know that you had to leave us early.
They all want you back,
and me too.

But the magic of the screen
will have to stay on the screen.

Dick van Dyke can still dance
but you can't even breathe.
It just turned out that way.

So, you say, "Don't try to find me."
You don't want us to go to Disneyland
thinking of you, and how you designed
our routes through the park
and where we got our fast passes
and where you lost John David,
for two hours, when he was four.
You want us to *just go*.

You don't want us to think about the magic
that could bring you back—
but the thinking of you
we're going to keep.

We'll try to find you in everything
and sometimes we will and
sometimes we won't,
but no matter what you say
we will always try.

Thought Crimes

Sex is the first one
we puritans think of
but there are more,
and much worse,

as when we hate
our own country because of
the bombs that explode
in other countries,

when we find God's natural world on fire
and hear of people and animals that died—
we think less of Him,
then remember, we don't believe at all.

When our own dear friend dies young and
we know our own life without his jokes and company
is smaller and cheaper—we don't want to live
as much as we used to.

Shower Crying

I don't cry. Well,
maybe in the shower I might cry,
not sure.

In the shower, you don't know you're crying,
they don't know your crying
only God knows your crying.

Okay, now I remember,
I guess I do.
I car cry.

Others

The Navy Captain's House

The Navy Captain's house was not burning,
but the sprinklers were firing every second on top of
this house he retired to thirty years ago
with his wife, who takes many medications now,
and his infant daughter, now a mother.

> Fifty years before, cruising with supplies from Guam,
> the Navy Captain heard his crew talking
> about the Japanese-made torpedoes that run swift and straight
> ten or twenty feet deep, anytime, piercing through the hull
> and exploding mostly inside the ship
> among the engines and the men.

He never thought he'd be safe at his daughter's house,
from the thoughts of the hundreds of homes already burned,
the news stations broadcasting no foreseeable containment,
and the fact that the fire had spread fingers
across Moraga Drive, the street just houses
from the Navy Captain's house.

> Standing on the deck at night, looking over the side,
> multiple straight lines glow the water to light,
> tracking amidships, making him think it is over.
> The Navy Captain grips the rail and bends his knees
> to see the South Pacific Dolphin turn to ride the bow
> of his destroyer.

He drank his bourbon, now a premature evacuee,
saying "If it goes, it goes... but Katherine will never recover from it."
We'll try to sleep tonight, call a neighbor in the morning,
the one with teenagers sitting on their roof watching the fire
surrounding the Navy Captain's house.

The Last Ringmaster

"The elephants are walking down main street!
We gotta go!"

The voice might as well have been Opey singing
"The Wells Fargo Wagon isa,
comin' down the street…"
through his missing two front teeth.

We went. Most of us went.
Whether P.T. Barnum was a cruel man at the time,
or just by today's standards a multi-species
slave owner, we went.

There's a man being shot
from a canon.
Those knives are just missing that lady
and really sticking in the board as she spins.
They make a convincing thud.
Are they coming from behind the board
or is that guy really throwing them?
Look up at that man walking a wire, with no net?

Tigers. Lions. And a person right there in the cage with them.
Evil by our standards, but on circus founder's day
in 1871, tailing on the Civil War,
it was kindness that animals were being fed
compared to what happened here among us,
and the reason we were burning each other's homes and crops.

But we have changed a bit, so an art form must die,

as if to give way to small screens that glow at night
in bed, keeping us awake, so we have to watch more
YouTubes actually recorded right while one car hits another.

We are kinder to animals, we say, while at the same time,
as animals, we plow and fertilize their jungles,
so they won't be here at all, anyway, but the debate is closed.

So, it falls to Jonathan Lee Iverson, the last ringmaster,
to announce the end of the circus on May 21, 2017, and
take that tightrope with him.

Again

Fire went into the roots
of the young, but dry, tree.
(A specimen whose ancestors
the Polynesians would cut
and smolder into coal.)

There weren't many trees
in the way of the fire,
(these trees that grew between the floes
of lava moon rock on the volcano slope)
and only a very strong wind
broke off a chunk of flame
that charred and smoldered
fragrant smoke thick and unbreathable.

The fire went into the roots,
the long roots that find no water,
that entwine with other roots,
other trees.

A thousand yards away, sixteen years later,
a connected tree bends for the wind,
creaks, explodes, and is consumed in orange burning.

Bait Ball

Small fish school tightly,
rise to flee feeding tuna
and find birds above.

Ocean Swimming

The most romantic thing I do
has nothing to do with a woman
but rather a swim in the Pacific Ocean.

I enter through the smooth waves
of the early morning, moisture surrounding me
and then my face, longing to be underneath,
completely inside,
to see the details, less dim,
in the bottom silt, small peaks
echo-waving water motion from the surface.

I flipper slowly watching the sea react to me,
the fish dart when I get too close,
a small ray on the bottom comes out of hiding,
shaking camouflage off its back
while it skittles naked, glides and then
shudders its small wings in a clouded stop
covering itself again,

the visual indicator of the ocean's orgasm
and retreat to modesty.

Summary of a S.F. Chronicle article by George Snyder,
Chronicle North Bay Bureau

Diver Tells How Shark Bit His Head

Only minor wounds in attack
at beach on Sonoma Coast

An abalone diver was recovering at home yesterday
after he was attacked and mauled Saturday
by a shark in waters off Jenner.

Rodney Orr, an electrician and part-time commercial fisherman,
was attacked by what appeared to be a great white shark
while he was diving near isolated rocks
at Russian Gulch Beach.

"My head was in its mouth" he said,
"I could see the teeth at an angle."

"It was a really frightening experience,"
Orr said.

"You think you know what is going to happen to you,
but then you really don't."

The Suitor's Room

The Alpha Phi House had a suitor's room. Liz came downstairs, dressed nicely, and met me there. This was our fifth date. It was time to tell her. It would be over, but it was my fate. I knew the trade someone made on my behalf, behind some curtain or during anesthesia, was an agreement directly with the devil. The chemotherapy would sterilize me, but I would live.

What if she thought of children, frequently, our children, the ones that would never be? What if, when I did tell her, she felt betrayed, threw her wine in my face, ran off crying?

So, it was time.

"Liz, there's something we need to talk about. Among the treatments, the MOPP chemotherapy sterilized me."

There was a pause as her emotionless face looked back at me through the dim light of the suitor's room.

"I know. I looked it up weeks ago."

Acknowledgments

The *Ocean State Review*, Charles Kell editor, was the first to publish "The Sweater" in their 2016 edition.

"The Rest of Them" was first published in *JAMA Oncology*, one of the journals of the American Medical Association, in August of 2017.

All the Bridgehampton poems were published in my book, *Bridgehampton*, as well as journals, described below.

> "Road-Side Farm Stand," "Sweet Corn" and "Mecox Beach" were all published in 2017 in the online *Scene and Heard Journal*.

> "The Light," and "The Geese," were published online by *Open Thought Vortex*, for their "Father Time" theme, in January of 2018, Kara Post-Kennedy editor. They were published again in 2020 by the *Monterey Poetry Review* in their September edition.

"Havana Club" and "No Religion" were published in 2018 by *Wanderlust Journal*.

Kingdoms in the Wild was the first to publish "Between the Mangroves."

The haiku "Everyday" was first published in *Smeuse* Poetry, a print anthology, in 2017.

The Scene and Heard Journal published "The Lover's Etiquette" and the photograph "A Young Rose" for their Valentine's Web Edition in 2018.

Alternating Currents accepted "Love Locks" for their publication, *The Coil*, in June of 2020.

"He Likes Primary Colors," was published on September 21, 2019 in the *Showbear Family Circus*. http://lanceschaubert.org/2019/09/21/he-likes-primary-colors/

"He Takes Chances" was published online by the *Remembered Arts Journal* in the summer of 2019.

All the Heavenly Whispers poems were published in my book, *Heavenly Whispers*, as well as the journal and anthology described below.

> The medical journal *CHEST* first published "Heavenly Whispers," the title poem of my book of the same name, in July of 2017.

> "The Neighbor Lady" was first published in the 2017 *Bacopa Literary Review* annual collection.

"Kissing on the Cliff" was first published by *Her Heart Poetry* in July of 2017.

"So Many Stars" was first published online in June of 2017 by *Open Thought Vortex*, Kara Post-Kennedy editor.

"To Walk with Laura" was first published by the *Ocean State Review*, 2018 Edition, Charles Kell editor.

The poem trilogy "Cattle" was first published in *Alternating Currents Footnote #4* edition in the Spring of 2020.

The Literary Nest published "The Navy Captain's House" in their Winter 2017/2018 issue, themed as their "Fear" edition.

Young Ravens Literary Review was the first to publish "The Last Ringmaster" in its *Issue 7* in 2017.

The Magnolia Review was the first to publish "Again" in their February 2018 edition, which had a theme of "fire."

The Poetry Box accepted "Ocean Swimming" for publication in a print anthology with a sports theme in 2019.

"Diver Tells How Shark Bit His Head" was published in the *Tiny Seed Journal*, an online nature-focused fine arts blog, on January 8, 2021.

Acknowledgments

"The Suitor's Room" won the monthly flash fiction prize from *Two Sister's Writing and Publishing* and was published on their web site in March of 2019 and will be in their anthology for 2020.

"Shower Crying" was almost a dictation from rambling comments made by Dave's daughter, Kathleen Langlais, while she was driving me in my dingy from the boat to the shore during cocktail hour in Avalon Harbor, Catalina Island. My wife is her God Mother, so she calls me her God Father, even though I am quite the atheist.

In the Extra Years